Overcomer

*Rising Above the Challenges of
Poland Syndrome*

Melissa Amaya

Book Layout © 2014 BookDesignTemplates.com

Overcomer / Melissa Amaya -- 1st ed.
ISBN 978-1512336115

Dedicated to my children:

Abigail, Annabella, Alexander and Austin.

May I be a better mother due to the experiences that are contained in this book.

CONTENTS

Preface

Why am I writing?

I make no claim to be any sort of authority on the issues of affliction and suffering; many have suffered much greater than I. At this very moment a friend comes to mind who deals with debilitating asthma, which often leaves her hospitalized and requires endless medical concoctions that doctors only hope will help. I suspect she is often frustrated with her physical limitations and the effect it has on her family. So am I the end-all on the topic of struggle? Hardly. But I have found that help and comfort don't always come from the experts. Often hope is offered through the every-day person, one who has walked through the same trials and struggles and is now a few steps ahead. Today, I may be that every-day person, walking a few steps ahead of you.

There are a variety of intentions and reasons for writing this book. For one, it is a type of therapy for me. I started this book years ago and the initial outline has been collecting dust in an old salt and pepper notebook for some time. Putting thoughts on paper has always helped me deal with problems, make decisions, and make sense of situations. Secondly, and equally important, I hope this book will help at least one person to: deal with a problem, find comfort in knowing that others have faced similar struggles, or learn about a world foreign to them, so that their judgment and confusion is transformed into understanding and compassion.

I enjoy anonymity. I dislike being the center of any sort of fuss or attention, negative or positive. My husband and I eloped partly because the thought of walking down the aisle, with all eyes on me, made me break out into cold sweats. I dislike being noticed. As I sit at my computer and type these words, in the back of my mind I wonder how far these words will travel? Who will know? If the people I personally know read this book, will that make things weird? (Probably not for them, but for me, most likely). As I go through life, part of my wish is that my condition will not be an issue, not a talking point, and in some ways, not even acknowledged. In other words, I desire to be *normal* and to be treated *normally*.

So why, then, would I write and allow others to read my deepest, most vulnerable thoughts? Well, strangely enough, I have little pause at the thought of strangers reading. What does make me uncomfortable is the possibility of those strangers becoming acquaintances. In a twisted way of processing, I don't mind people knowing, I just don't want to talk about it. And if the people that know are the people that know *me,* then there is the potential of them wanting to talk about it. Nevertheless, I feel compelled in a way. I know that God works all things for good (Romans 8:28), and that He ordains everything that takes place. He knitted me together (Psalm 139:13), Poland Syndrome and all. He has a purpose for everything He does, and therefore He has a purpose for my

Poland Syndrome. As I look back on my past, I can see some definite purposes for my PS, which I will explain.

But are God's purposes for this limited to my past? I believe God answered that for me as I was reading my Bible recently. In Philippians 1:12-13 Paul talks about God's purpose for his current situation. He was in jail, but not because he stole from someone or murdered someone. No, he was in jail simply because he went about the towns telling people about Jesus Christ. It was an unjust imprisonment and from a human perspective he had every right to whine and complain. But he didn't see it that way. Due to His imprisonment, the whole imperial guard heard the Gospel, and for that he rejoiced. Paul was afflicted for the sake of the Gospel. Could the same be true of me?[1]

So, despite not being a very open person when it comes to my personal life, I decided to let my guard down and share my very personal, and very guarded story because there is a possibility that it may help you. Everything you read will be from my heart in as pure and honest manner as possible. I hope you enjoy the journey through my story.

---

[1] I recognize that as you read, you may not be a Christian. You may even be an atheist. This is not a "Christian" book, per se. Please do not put this down simply because of the mentioning of the Bible here. My desire is to reach anyone and everyone that has been effected by PS, regardless of religion, and the content of this book is applicable to you, regardless of religion.

{ 1 }

A Brief Explanation of Poland Syndrome

Most likely you picked up this book because you have a direct connection with Poland Syndrome. Maybe you have PS and are trying to cope with the struggles. Or, perhaps, you are comfortable in your own skin, but are interested in knowing the story of a fellow PS-er. Or maybe you are new parents, your precious baby has Poland Syndrome, and you are overwhelmed with questions, concerns and heartaches right now.

Perhaps you are the parent of an older child, even an adult child with PS, and want a glimpse into what your child may have endured growing up. For you, the information here may be redundant. There may be others of you, over-achieving friends or family, who simply know someone with PS, and want to better understand them and their affliction. For you, the information in this chapter may be new.

There may be a third group of people with no connection to Poland Syndrome, but rather a connection to another condition. Your interest here may be in the realm of afflictions in general. For you, this chapter may also be helpful.

All that to say, if this is old-news for you, I won't be offended if you skip ahead; I won't even know.

Poland What?

"Poland what?" is the usual response I get when I begin to explain this condition. I want to keep this book as non-technical as possible, but I feel that in order to understand my struggles, and the struggles of others with PS, an adequate amount of background information about P.S. is needed.

Poland Syndrome is also known as Poland Anomaly and Poland Sequence. It is a rare medical condition that results in a physical deformity of the hand and chest on one side of the body.[2] The severity of the affliction varies drastically from case to case. Some folks are only effected in the hand, some only in the chest. Some also have a shortened arm, or missing ribs on the effected side. The severity of the malformation of the hand varies as well. Some have stubbed digits, others lack up to three digits. The chest deformity includes the lack of the pectoral major muscle and in some cases the pectoral minor muscle as well. In males, the visual effect is a concave pectoral muscle on the effected side; in females, it results in a

---

[2] 1 in 20,000 people are effected. Poland's Syndrome is three times more common in boys than girls, and effects the right side of the body twice as often as the left. The reasons and cause for these differences are unknown.

retarded growth or a total lack of growth in the effected breast.

In my case, I have a total lack of growth in the right breast and a deformed right hand. When I was born I had two semi-normal looking digits (pinkie and thumb) and three stubs in between. Today, post hand-surgery, I have two digits whose growth was quite stunted and scars in between from the removal of the three stubs. My right hand is somewhat functional – similar to a claw. I can grasp most things, as long as they are not too heavy.

{ 2 }

Snapshots of Struggle

Having any kind of disability creates a multi-faceted effect on life. Physical deformities obviously cause physical struggles and require adaptation, but that is only one aspect of having a disability. If also touches the emotional, social, and even spiritual aspects of life to one degree or another. I offer here a few snapshots of how Poland Syndrome touched various aspects of my life while growing up, with the hope that it will provide some context for information shared later in this book.

Learning to Adapt

Much of my life can de defined by the word *adaptation*. From my earliest days, I was challenged to adapt so that I could function like a normal kid. In a lot of ways it was fun: fun to figure things out, fun to find a way to do what other kids did, fun to exceed expectations and do what others thought I couldn't do. My dedication to adapting was clearly evidenced by my early determination to master the monkey bar rings.

When you have only one fully functioning hand, the rings seem impossible, but my early childhood was one long feat of seeking to do the "impossible". I discovered that if I extended my arm through the ring, grasping it with the cleft of my elbow, I could propel myself forward enough to then grasp the next ring with my "good" left hand. I (quietly) took pride in this accomplishment, and the broken blood vessels on my arm were my war scars after recess each day. I gloried in this achievement on a daily basis throughout elementary school.

Delicate Balance

Growing up, part of me wanted to fit in enough to be invisible. I wanted to be just like everyone else. I did not want any attention because of my hand. At the same time, I possessed a quiet arrogance that allowed me to cover up any insecurity regarding my hand. Soccer was my best example of that quiet arrogance.

I excelled in soccer and, through my years of schooling, it served as a mask, allowing me to avoid dealing with the issues of having Poland's Syndrome. In elementary school, I was the only girl allowed to play soccer with the boys at recess. (They didn't have much of a choice since I was better than all but two of them). On the soccer field, my hand did not matter. My foot skills took all attention off of my physical imperfections and I loved that. I could "wow" any spectator and gain the positive feedback that fed my ego, masked my pain, and filled the hole PS created, all at the same time.

I've Got Your Back

The innocence of young kids is a wonderful thing. I never had to explain myself to friends. I never had to justify myself or explain my hand. Friends never asked. They just accepted me…and they had my back.

One day on the playground a boy decided to pick on me with disparaging comments about my hand. A good friend, Kristine, didn't miss a beat in speaking up for me and shutting the boy down. It felt so good to not have to justify myself. To have this friend stand by my side, speak up on my behalf, and refuse to allow me to be picked on provided a great sense of security.

Good Intentions…But No Thank You

I often found the good intention of others to be unwanted. As a youngster, my grandmother made me custom fit mittens one year. As I opened the gift all my little mind could think was, "Oh great, lets draw more attention to my hand." Her intention was pure. She was trying to give a thoughtful gift and she spent her own time to make it. I appreciated that fact, but the gift itself was not appreciated. What made anyone think that I would want such a gift? It seemed to me both then and now that if anyone actually paid attention and took the time to know my thoughts, they would definitively know that such a gift would be the last thing I would find encouraging.

Another time we were at a family get-together at an Aunt's house. I was in the middle of wresting with my brother and two cousins (I was a bit of a tom-boy if you haven't caught on yet), when my mother called me over. She was talking to a woman we were somehow related to and this woman also had a deformed hand. I do not recall whether it was PS or another deformity, but my mother, for some reason, thought I might find it interesting to speak with this woman. What was she thinking? Did she know me at all? I wanted to crawl under a rock. The last thing I wanted, and the last thing I still want, is someone drawing attention to my hand. I tried to be polite and sought to return to the wrestling match as quickly as possible.

More Fun with Problem Solving

Having any kind of physical deformity can make life quite interesting. I was a Girl Scout in elementary school. We once took a field trip that introduced us to a variety of handicap issues. We got to try out a wheel chair – that was fun. We spoke with a man who had an artificial arm, which wow-ed all of us.

But more than those two events, one aspect of this trip particularly stuck with me. At one station in this center we put on rubber gloves and tried some basic dexterity tasks. The purpose was to show us how difficult these basic tasks were to certain people who had a particular issue. I do not recall the name of the disease or affliction, but I do remember the effect this had on me.

At each of the stations we each got to "try on" these different handicaps, but with this particular station the trip was no longer pretend, no longer an experiment in stepping into someone else's shoes. Instead, it was a reminder of my own handicap. Dexterity issues are something I deal with every day of my life. Some seemingly simple tasks aren't so simple. And since having children, the list of those tasks is growing.

I studied Karate for many years, and when I reached the stage of learning weapons, my Sensei was stretched in her ability to help me adapt. During weapons class, as we shifted from Bo to Sai, the first five minutes were spent taping me up. I had no ability to manipulate the Sai with my right hand, so we would tape it to my arm. Then we had to figure out how to adjust the Kata to accommodate the stationary Sai. My left side would do the Kata as normal, extending and retracting the Sai as needed. My right side continuously had the Sai retracted against my arm.

Dealing with my hand in this context never caused self-consciousness. I'm not sure I can pinpoint why. It was what it was, we dealt with it, and we moved on. My hand wasn't going away and new issues would always arise, requiring more adaptation. As long as I could deal with the issue without my hand becoming a permanent focal point, I felt as close to "normal" as possible.

Another sports context that required some problem solving involved a tool called the Reaction Coach. My brother and I began working with a soccer trainer to improve our fitness and speed. The trainer utilized this particular machine to quicken our reaction time. To use it we had to hold a baton in each hand. We would move in a particular direction and hit a particular target with the baton. The sound produced would register our speed.

My right hand was not strong enough to hold the baton securely. At first my solution was to use my left hand by reaching across my body and hitting the target on the right. It worked, but the it resulted in an inaccurate speed. I soon discovered that I could use my watch. I used the band of the watch to secure the baton to my arm, providing the additional support needed to hold it steady. Problem solved! To this day, 15 years later, I still remember the reaction of the trainer when he saw my solution. Surprising people never gets old.

These are some of the fun challenges from life, but there are plenty of mundane challenges that are downright annoying. I remember standing in front of my bedroom door, trying over and over again to grasp and turn the doorknob with my right hand, a daily task that I suspect most people take for granted. I was tired of always having to use my left hand and was determined to figure it out. I did finally get the hang of it, but not without pain. The mental concentration was draining and the awkward movement whole arm had to undergo to open the door left me in pain.

There are still some doors that I cannot open because they are too heavy or the knob too tight. And to this day I can still get frustrated with myself for my inability to open certain doors. Some challenges never go away.

{ 3 }

Getting to the Heart of the Matter

Without realizing it, I had created a wall of protection around me in the form of athletics. I excelled at sports, receiving many accolades. As long as I was playing sports, mainly soccer in my teen years, I could put all worries aside, including any reminder of my PS. On the field, my hand made no difference, no one noticed, no one cared. I could dribble and kick a ball pretty well, and that's all that mattered.

After high school I went off to the University of Pennsylvania to study business and play soccer. My love for the game had been dwindling the last few years and after my first season at Penn I quit the team. That's when I realized that soccer had been my wall of protection all those years. Without the idol of sport, my world came crashing down. I went into an 18-month depression and, without my safeguard, finally faced the effects PS had on me.

Melissa Amaya

The "Why" Question

I was forced to ask myself some tough questions. I needed to evaluate who I was, without soccer. Soccer always defined me, so without soccer, what was my purpose?

I began asking myself, "Why me?" And was surprised at the answer. I had gone through my share of pity parties in my life, but eventually came an encouraging conclusion.

PS led to extreme self-consciousness with my body. I never wanted to be "found out," especially during those years when we all feel awkward enough without any additional challenges. I could only imagine the taunts if certain boys learned of how the condition effected my chest. Once I started developing, I was lopsided until I underwent the process of reconstructive surgery and even then I could notice a difference.

But at a time when most of my friends were playing with sex, I abstained. My inner conscience told me it was wrong, but peer pressure can be a powerful thing. Thankfully, for me, peer pressure was no match for my self-consciousness. So my PS kept me pure at a time and in an environment that caused many of my friends to fall.

I was grateful for this and as a college student looking back I could see how PS had served a wonderful purpose. But what now? I made it through high school pure, where almost 50% of folks have sex before graduating. As a 19 year old peer pressure in this area no longer had an effect on me.

But now my thoughts turned to something more long term. What about marriage? Would any guy be interested in me if he knew? And how in the world was I going to get past my insecurities in general and let down my guard enough to get to know a guy anyway? The walls I created served their purpose well, but how do I go about breaking down those walls now?

Such Irony

I was attending one of the top business schools in the nation, yet I hated one of the fundamental marks of a confident businessperson, a firm handshake. How am I supposed to shake someone's hand when I have half a hand? I remember debating in my head many times over the years whether I would have preferred my PS to be on the left side rather then that right (as if I had a choice). My reasoning went like this, with my right hand deformed, handshakes pose a problem, but if it were my left hand, then if/when I got married, placement of my wedding ring would be an issue. I could always put the ring on the other hand, but that might draw attention to the deformity.

Three Categories of People

I often place people into one of three categories based upon how they shake my hand. I rarely (1 in 100 rarely) extend my hand first. It is such an uncomfortable feeling for me to have my hand out there, awaiting the other person. There are many times when I wish I didn't have this reaction.

I am certain that I can come across as cold when I meet people because of my hesitancy to extend a hand, our American symbol of friendship. But I just cannot get over that fear, and my three categories of people may explain why.

I'll start with my least favorite, the folks I dread. I'll call this category the "jumpers." These jumpers, upon making palm-to-palm contact, jerk their hand away, or even literally jump back, in reaction to this strange thing they touched. I understand it to be a knee-jerk reaction, not a premeditated act, yet that knowledge helps very little when you are the recipient of such a reaction. Don't be this person. I will sometimes get an "I'm sorry" after they pull themselves together.

The next category is a step up, and I am perfectly fine with these folks. I'll call them the "lookers." The lookers, upon that palm-to-palm contact, look down at my hand and then look back up, continuing the shake. Sometimes there is a pause in the shaking when they look, sometimes not.

I am very aware that my hand is different. I am very aware that 99.9% of the people I meet will never have met someone with PS. So when they touch my hand curiosity is bound to arise. The lookers do just that, they look. They want to see why the hand feels different, and once they do, they move on. No apology is ever offered here, none is needed.

While the lookers are quite fine, my favorite category is the "shakers." They just shake my hand, no jumping, no flinching, no looking. They grab hold, as they would anyone else, and give no notice to anything different. For obvious reasons, I feel most comfortable in these encounters. The hand is a non-issue for them, which allows me to make it a non-issue in interacting with them.

I've encountered one person in my life that falls outside of all three categories here. She meant well, but for me, I'd prefer she just join the lookers or the shakers.

In college I was pledging in a business fraternity (how nerdy can you get). This was a co-ed fraternity that was business oriented. Part of the pledging process involved interviews with the brothers (both men and women). I went in for my interview rather nervous, hoping they liked me. The meeting was with two of them, a fellow (who I forget) and a German woman who held some of the typical German stereotypes; a little uptight, staunch, and curt. She was a bit intimidating, so I was not looking forward to the interview.

I entered the room and, knowing that a business fraternity is looking for business-minded folks, I forced myself to extend my hand. Well, she and I extended our hands at the same time and to my surprise she extended her left hand. I suppose through the interactions leading up to this point, she noticed my hand. In attempt to show respect, or compassion, or something, she sought to shake my good hand. I really did appreciate the gesture, especially coming from her, but I kept my right hand out on principle until we did a proper shake.

It was a new experience for me then and I really didn't know what to do. I would probably handle it differently today. I suspect I would just switch and extend my left. I am *slightly* more comfortable in my own skin now and would be better able to laugh it off.

Handshakes

At some point in business school someone taught me how to do a proper handshake. Be the first to extend. Make it firm, but not a killer grip. Don't shake too hard. Know when to let go. All I wanted to do was whine, "But what if I don't want to?"

Prior to starting college I never thought about how my aversion to handshakes might effect my business career. I'm not talking about discrimination because of my hand, but rather my hesitancy to shake hands says something about me. Unfortunately, the message it portrays is not the message I want to portray nor is it accurate. Nevertheless, we are often judged, in any arena, by first impressions and a hearty handshake is part of that first impression for business people.

A few years ago I started a consulting business where much of my time was spent on the sales end. Once again, I never considered how my aversion to handshakes would set the tone here. I got into sales meetings, knowing that I need to introduce myself, thank them for their time, and shake their hand. But I don't want to. What a great first impression I give. I often wonder how much more of a people person I might be if I could give a hearty handshake, without any hesitancy, when I meet new people.

Don't Touch My Hand

Handshakes are just one form of hand touching that I dislike. I have never liked people touching my hand. In elementary school, the "Okay everyone, lets hold hands and make a circle" game would cause me to sweat. Even someone brushing my hand on accident would cause me to instinctively pull my arm away.

In college, after those fraternity interviews I mentioned above, a friend who was also pledging was recounting to me her experience with the scary German woman. This was a friend I played soccer with. She knew me pretty well, and definitely knew about my hand. She was showing me how the German woman shook her hand in a rather overeager way.

Without warning, my friend grabbed my right hand and reenacted her experience, she as the German woman and I as her. As usual my initial thought was about her touching my hand, and I was half-expecting some kind of reaction on her part when she realized what she had done and what kind of hand she was shaking. That moment never came and I quickly realized she didn't care. I didn't faze her one bit. Here I was, practically hyperventilating over something that was of no concern to her. That was refreshing.

Let Me Be Invisible

During my senior year of high school,I got my first job – at Pizza Hut. It wasn't glamorous, but it was a job and it earned (some) money. I enjoyed being gainfully employed so it's a shame it didn't last longer than two weeks.

My job was in the kitchen making the pizza. I would take the pre-made crust and build the pizza with sauce and the desired toppings. I'd put the pizza in one side of the conveyor oven and remove it on the other side. Removing the pizza was harder than it sounds as it took a bit of strength and some balance. The pizza tray was hot, obviously, so it was a two-handed procedure. One hand would use a plier-like tool to grasp the rim of the tray and the other hand would place a spatula under the tray to support the weight of it while I brought it to the counter to cut. This was by far the most difficult aspect of the job for me, but also the most fun, because I always love a challenge.

Almost two weeks into the job, I was removing a pizza from the oven when one of my coworkers (finally) noticed my hand. She was impressed with my ability to handle the pizza despite my hand. A small part of me appreciated her comment, but most of me just wanted to be anonymous. I wasn't looking for any kind of acknowledgement. I simply wanted to enjoy the challenge and do my job without being made to feel "special" or "different" or in any way exceptional for simply doing my job. But alas, that was about to end.

Within an hour my boss (a very large man) called me into the walk-in cooler. There, he gave me a most unnecessary and most unwelcome monologue of advice. I suppose that coworker went to the boss and told him of my hand. That is the only logical explanation for what was said.

He proceeded to lecture me on how it's okay that my hand is the way it is. He said something to the effect of, "I'm fat (he was very obese), and you have a different hand, I'm okay, you're okay." I couldn't get out of there fast enough. I was mortified. All I could think was, "What in the world? What did I do or say to encourage this?"

I quit the very next day.

While I suppose he intended to be helpful or encouraging, I was downright offended. And there was no way I wanted to work for a person who took such liberty to address something that was none of his business. I was also offended by the comparison he made. Which brings me to another aspect of well-intended pity.

Don't Compare

This man had the audacity (can you tell that I'm still bothered by the incident?) to compare by birth-deformed hand with his obesity. There was little to nothing in common between the two. My situation was imposed upon me, the way I was created, totally out of my control. His condition was a result of eating too much for too long[3]. This wasn't the only time that a well-intentioned person made a comparison that didn't sit well with me.

That same year, I opened up to a friend for the first time about PS and some of my struggles. I was sharing my concern over shaking people's hands, and the self-consciousness involved. She then shared her own insecurities with me. I can see that divulging her own private struggle was a leap of faith, but at the time it echoed the comparison my boss made.

As I shared self-consciousness about a (rather rare, given from birth) physical deformity; she shared with me her self-consciousness over her height and weight. This was not a fat girl. She was an athlete. We played soccer and basketball together in middle school and high school, and she also played lacrosse. Fat was not an adjective that anyone would have used to describe her, yet it was something she thought about. And height, well, she was indeed 'vertically challenged,' and was often teased for it, in what most thought was a harmless manner.

While I did not want to do anything to belittle her own areas of struggle, I was not receiving her well intended comparison in the way she intended and all I could think was, "This is not the same." Yet she couldn't see that.

---

[3] I recognize that some people may have a greater struggle with weight than others due to medical or genetic conditions. I am not making light of those struggles. However, even people in those situations do have a degree of control over their weight, whereas someone with a deformity has no ability to change that condition. Aside from that, this man's obesity was a result of eating Pizza Hut every day for 20+ years, regardless of any genetic issues he may have had.

How many short people do you know? How many folks with a physical deformity do you know? That was the thought in my head at that moment. Her attempt to console me was failing because her comparison was not an accurate one and therefore not helpful. Being short is common, and *short* is a relative term anyway. But having a malformed hand isn't so common. The average short person lack of height won't cause people to literally jump back, but my hand has done so on many occasions.

{ 4 }

The Role Parents Can Play

It's one of the most exciting days of your life; maybe it's your first child, maybe your fifth. You just know that a precious child will be placed in your arms today for you to raise and care for. The baby arrives and when doctor takes inventory, the count for ten fingers and ten toes comes up short.

Or perhaps the count does reach ten, but fast forward ten or eleven years when your child is entering puberty. You notice your daughter isn't developing evenly, or your son's muscle structure doesn't quite seem right.

In either of these scenarios, you are no doubt crushed, with a million questions racing through your head. What in the world are you to do? Thankfully, we live in a digital age, and as you have found my book, you can find other resources to help you through this.

But the question stands, what can parents do?

I stand here today at 29 years old. I have the ability to look back on what my folks did and didn't do. With hindsight, I can see what was helpful and what wasn't. I am also a mom to four (one still in the oven), as of the writing of this book, so I carry the perspective of living with PS, but also the foresight of what I might do if one of my children are born with PS.

I remember one of my OB visits during my first pregnancy. While taking my blood, the doctor's assistant asked if I was worried about my child having PS. My response was a quick and definitive "No," but the answer isn't that easy.

Ask an expectant parent whether they want a boy or a girl and they might answer with, "It doesn't matter as long as they have 10 finger and 10 toes." So what do you do when your child doesn't arrive quite as perfectly as expected?

So how do I answer the question, "Am I worried about my child having PS?"

If the question is, 'Am I grateful for the lessons I've learned through this affliction?" The answer is "Yes." Am I thankful for the way that trials have made me a stronger person? Or course. Would I want my child to grow as I have? Absolutely. But would I pick this way for them to learn those lessons? No.

Thankfully, it's not my decision. The Lord will decide what is best and will work all things for good.

The one advantage I have if a child with PS or another physical deformity were to join our family is that I've already been there. I can relate a bit more than my folks could. What if my parents were given insight into what their daughter would experience, and knew how to better guide her? It is my hope to act as a guide of sorts, providing that first hand insight. I cannot guarantee that everything I say will apply to every scenario. Rather, as I sit here today, looking back on 29 years of life, I set out to answer the question of what my parents could have done differently to better address the challenges of PS.

Let me make it clear, my folks did the best they could with what they knew. They did many things right, and I'm sure followed the best advice given to them at the time. They advocated on my behalf to ensure that I received the necessary surgeries to give me the best chance of having a functional hand. They fought with insurance companies in my teen years to get me reconstructive surgery for my chest. My parents were on my side, but unfortunately, intention does not always equate with wisdom.

So to the mom or dad who is reading:

Talk About It!

Don't make it the elephant in the room. I guarantee that PS is constantly in your child's thoughts, whether you talk about it or not. In my household, PS was not discussed. The silence made it clear that this was my battle. I was alone. In later years, as I began to undergo numerous reconstructive surgeries, my mom tried to enter that part of my life, and I shut her out. It was my battle before that, why should I trust her to enter that battle now?

I have only one memory from childhood of talking about PS with my family. (Please, parents don't let this be the case in your home.) I was getting into our family van. I was probably 10 or 11 at the time, and my brother was 5 or 6. He said to my mom, "Mom, why does Melissa only have 2 fingers on her hand." My mom gave him some sort of pat answer, and then asked me if I ever get asked about it at school. I quickly answered no, and that was it. That was the extent of any discussion I recall being initiated by my parents.

That is not good enough. PS should be a topic of conversation, like anything else. If you have a girl, conversation around her stunted breast growth would best be kept in a private setting with Mom for modesty reasons, obviously. But overall, this should not be a hush-hush issue. Otherwise, you are adding shame to something that should not shameful.

Ask First

Before you share with a friend, a relative, or anyone, ask your child first. This obviously does not apply to an infant, but as your child gets older, it is important that s/he has a say in what information is shared about him/her to others. I recall after my first reconstructive surgery, as I was recovering in bed, I was told I had a visitor.

I was in a lot of pain the first few days after surgery. I couldn't even adjust my position in bed without hurting. To hear that I had a visitor, after being unkempt, un-bathed, half-drugged and tired from not sleeping well, did not go over well. On top of that, this was a very private and shameful issue for me, so why would I want a visitor?

I turned out to be my Grandma. I'm sure my folks meant well, I'm sure Grandma wanted to make me feel better, but nobody asked me. Here I was in bed, wanting to be alone, yet there was a guest standing in my doorway.

Parents, brothers, sisters, and all others, **ask first**. Use direct and clear communication so that there are no misunderstandings and no hurt feelings. And after you ask, respect your child's wishes. It is about them, not you. It's about them, not whether a desire for privacy might offend Aunt Sally.

Your family is not entitled to know any details. You and your child may choose to share information with them, but do not allow family, under the guise of "concern," to guilt you into sharing information that is best kept private. This includes the extent of the condition and the treatment options (i.e. reconstructive surgery). Respect your child's wishes in how much information to share, when, and with whom.

Don't Coddle

While PS needs to be an open discussion, do not use it as an excuse to coddle your child. PS creates challenges, but it does not hinder any type of normal life with normal capabilities. There is no reason to have "special chores" for Johnny because his hand is deformed. Johnny still needs to learn to function in the world. His case may be so extreme that one hand is completely absent or useless. All that means is that Johnny will need to learn to adapt in order to succeed in life. That life training starts at home.

I am not suggesting you set your child up to fail. On the contrary, you always want to be giving age and ability appropriate chores, jobs, and expectations. That is true for any child, and PS may factor into that calculation. However, don't try to make life easier for Johnny by removing anything that may challenge or frustrate him, because when you do that, you are setting him up for failure in the future.

When you see Sally struggling to tie her shoe because of her hand, don't run right over and do it for her. Give her a chance to struggle and figure it out. You will be amazed at the ability of your child to think outside the box and solve problems. A little struggle is a good thing.

Help Them Think Properly

If you are fostering open communication, as I am suggesting, then it is inevitable that your child will come to you with a scenario that upsets you. You may want to scream "unfair" when you hear of Johnny getting picked on at school. Or you may want to do things for Sally when she shares that tying her shoe is really difficult. Your job, Mom, Dad, is to help your child process information properly. You have experience they don't have. You possess a perspective that only comes with age. Don't always seek to fix the problem, but rather help them walk through the problem.

Say Johnny is getting picked on and is being called names. Praise him for keeping his temper and for trusting you enough to share that information. Role-play with him; ask how can we handle this next time? What can Johnny say in response to the bully? You may eventually have to call the teacher or the principal, but don't make that the first response. Johnny will deal with difficult people all his life. He needs the skills to do so.

Say Sally cannot tie her shoe, after trying many times. Praise her for her perseverance; remind her that she is learning patience as she tries. Brainstorm yourself on how she might succeed. Offer suggestions. Sit with her as she tries, if that is helpful for her. Keep encouraging. Even if tying a shoe is never mastered, it's the lessons she learns while trying that are important. And then, there is always Velcro for adults!

Beware of Comparisons

As I mentioned earlier, I have had some well-intentioned people in my life make comparisons between PS and their situation. The two examples I gave were comparisons that were not helpful. Even today with the benefit of hindsight, while I see their intention, I still find the comparisons unhelpful. And while not all comparisons are unhelpful, think carefully before you offer them.

When I was 15, in the months leading up to my first reconstructive surgery, I had lunch with my club soccer coach. This woman was a wonderful mentor in my life and will forever have a fond place in my heart. I was facing this surgery right after finishing up a very successful summer of soccer tournaments. (Part of me did not want to have the surgery; actually, most of me. Yet, in my strange thinking, it was easier to go along with the surgery because then I did not have to talk about it. If I had told my parents I did not want the surgery, it would have required a lengthy conversation about everything, which terrified me.)

So, I was facing this surgery, which would mean six weeks without training for soccer or even running. At this time I was at my peak physically, and six weeks off was the last thing I wanted. At this point, my coach was the only person with whom I had shared any details about the surgery and my condition.

We were having lunch and she was joking with me, trying to lighten the mood by asking if my doctor knew how much work we had put in over the summer. I didn't take her humor too well, and I think she sensed I needed some encouragement about the whole thing. So changing gears slightly, she shared with me that when she was a youth, she was also concerned about developing. Her concern was hoping that it didn't get in the way of playing sports.

For me, this *was* a helpful conversation. It still wasn't a perfect comparison to my scenario, but at least it was in the same realm of experience, and it did bring comfort and encouragement.

Every person is different. No doubt your child will have a different thought process than me in one way or another, so I am not advising that you see this as a prescription of what to do and what not to do. Rather, recognize that your best efforts may not be helpful, and before you offer what you consider great advice, think it through. Once you decide to offer that advice, do it with a great deal of gentleness and humility, recognizing that your son or daughter may not find it helpful or encouraging. Be willing to state that upfront, 'Johnny, I don't know if this is helpful at all, but…' After offering the advice ask, 'do you think that might work?' or whatever follow-up question fits the scenario. This will create greater dialogue and show your child a commitment on your part to help them with the struggle.

Change the Question

You need to be direct and intentional with your questions. Do not ask, "Does your hand ever cause you to struggle?" Instead ask, "What struggles do you have with your hand?" The struggles are there, you know it, so acknowledge it with your question. The second question forces an answer where the first allows them to say "No" to avoid talking about it. The following are some questions you may find helpful – tailor them to the age of your child:

- What is the biggest struggle you face due to PS?
- When was the last time you were picked on because of your hand?
- Do I (mom/dad) ever do/say anything that makes you self-conscious about your hand/PS?
- Do your siblings ever do/say anything that makes you self-conscious about your hand/PS?
- What have you learned from having to deal with PS?

- What's your neatest trick? (rephrase this to fit your child. Whenever I came up with an alternative way to do something, like open a door, I considered them tricks. I had a great sense of pride in accomplishing such things, and I suspect your child does too. Don't always make life with PS a negative thing, allow him/her to take pride in what s/he can accomplish.)

Is it Too Late?

If your child is already 6, or 16, you may need to sit down and admit that while you have done the best you can do, you know you have made many mistakes. Let them know that you found this resource, maybe even have them read it. Let them know that you are trying to learn more to better help them. If they are old enough to read this book, ask them to highlight parts that resonate with them. It may spark a conversation where they feel comfortable to share their struggles.

Your child doesn't need a perfect parent, but an honest and humble parent. It goes a long way for them to see your heart, to see your desire to do better. Your child knows that you don't know the details of their struggle, and that is okay. But if you are humbly seeking to understand them and their struggles, that will make them feel loved and secure.

Siblings

Encourage siblings to rally around your PS child. Siblings should always be each other's support, but even more so when an issue like this exists. Kids can be brutal, and siblings can help deflect the blows their brother or sister may endure.

Siblings need to be the biggest encouragers. If you have boys, tap into the innate desire to protect. If you have girls, foster their nurture instinct as they care for that sibling when s/he is struggling.

Foster open communication between your children. Your children should always feel welcome to ask a question. Especially the younger ones, who begin to notice differences and wonder why. The atmosphere of your home needs to be one in which those children know they can ask a "why" question, without being hushed. The younger the child, the more sincere you know the question is, because children have a wonderful lack of guile. They shoot straight.

Keep Things in Perspective

Above all, don't freak out. While it may feel like it, PS is really not the end of the world. Think about this, while your child will live with PS the rest of his/her life, s/he will LIVE. This is not a terminal illness. You child will not die due to PS. While this condition does effect so many aspects of life and creates a number of challenges, those challenges can be overcome.

Dad, She Needs You

Dads, do not underestimate the importance of your role in all this, especially if you have a girl. You may think that your wife has the more important role because of the female issues that she will face; but in many ways you, Dad, have the more important role. And that may be true for any daughter, whether or not she has PS.

Your daughter needs you. Her confidence as a young lady rests largely on your shoulders. I hope you feel the weight of that sentence, because it is a great responsibility. Thankfully, it is rather easy to fulfill.

She needs to know that you love her, just the way she is. She needs to know that you think she is beautiful, just the way she is. She needs unconditional love and affection from you, as a little girl, as a pre-teen, and as an adolescent. Every girl goes through awkwardness as they begin to develop. Your little girl will have additional awkwardness, as her development may be stunted or uneven. This can create a tremendous amount of anxiety and self-consciousness.

She craves male affirmation of who she is, and her first choice to get that affirmation is from you. If she fails to get that affirmation from you, she will seek it elsewhere. Dads, you were once a 13-year-old boy, do you really want your daughter getting that affirmation from him, given the thoughts that go through his mind daily?

{ 5 }

For the Girls

Depending on the severity of the PS, girls face some unique challenges. I have no doubt that the guys deal with their own self-consciousness. Most boys, as they hit adolescence especially, begin to mind their physique. Strength training often becomes important and "looking the part" is a priority. So for guys with PS who are missing the pectoral muscle, you will have to overcome your own struggles. I am aware that those struggles are real, but I am not about to presume to understand the male mind and the social pressure men face. I do, however, understand the pressures women face.

Unique Struggle

Going through puberty is tough enough without any additional issues; the awkwardness of bodies changing, hormones raging, and wondering where one fits into the social scene. It's a tough time. For a girl facing puberty with PS, utter dread may indeed be the proper adjective. I know it was for me.

As I have mentioned, my family did not talk about PS when I was growing up. As I reached the teen years, I do recall a time or two when my mom mentioned that one day I would have surgery on my breast to correct my PS. I never questioned it, but I don't know that I ever actually responded. I didn't want to talk about it. As an athlete, everything in life was filtered through the question of whether X will effect soccer. All in all, I was not looking forward to any kind of surgery.

The day came when the topic was broached in a more definitive manner. I was traveling home from somewhere with my mom, just she and I. We stopped off to eat something and she stated that she thought it was time I "see a specialist."

At first, I thought she was talking about getting a personal trainer for soccer, as my dad and I had a conversation to that effect just a few days before. With that in mind I quickly responded, "Yeah, Dad already talked to me about that." Once the issue was clarified, however, I just wanted to sink into a hole.

I had such mixed feelings about the whole concept of surgery and, to some degree, I still do. On the one hand, I didn't want to appear any different from others, so having surgery was a logical step. It would fill in my right side, where my breast would not naturally grow. On the other hand I wondered if it was vain to even care what others thought.

Shortly after this chat an appointment was made to meet with a cosmetic surgeon. Thankfully, we hit gold on the first try. We chatted with the doctor, who was familiar with PS, and seemed totally comfortable and at ease with the whole scenario. He took me into an exam room where one of the office workers helped him to set up. He inspected my breasts and took photos for the file. Despite being pleased with the physician, this was the beginning of feeling like a carnival freak show.

I left that appointment with my mom confident that this was the doctor I wanted to work with. His demeanor completely put me at ease. His office staff was wonderful, and I would come to look forward to my appointments. In a strange way, it was an opportunity to address the PS, even without having to talk about it.

The Start of Surgeries

I was 15 when I had the first surgery and, over the next three years, I would undergo four more (I think, I stopped counting at some point). This was a whole new experience for me: all the photos, the x-rays, the testing. I lost any sense of privacy over my body. I just went numb. It didn't have to be that way, but for me, it was. I remember going in to get a chest x-ray before my first surgery. My doctor wanted to see the skeletal frame of my torso, as PS often leads to missing ribs, which may effect the surgery.

In the hospital it was finally my turn. The technician told me to go behind a screen and remove my bra (I didn't know it was because bra underwire causes a problem to the x-ray machine. I always wore a sports bra, so this didn't apply to me). I just did as I was told and came out naked from the waist up. I quickly realized that was not what he meant. The shirt could stay, but the bra needed to come off. But at this point I didn't think anything of it. I felt so poked and prodded by now that standing in front of a stranger, half-naked for yet another medical thing didn't seem strange to me.

Despite the range of emotions I went through, my doctor really was amazing, as was his staff. Two women in particular made such a difference to me. I realize their job is to make patients feel comfortable, and I have no delusions to think that I was anything special to them. But they did their jobs well as I did feel comfortable. In a small way, every doctor visit was a small step in dealing with PS.

The Options and What to Expect

The people involved were wonderful, but surgery is still surgery. There is more than one option for how to deal with the breast abnormality. You need to find a good doctor who will go over all your options with you, but I'll share the course that I took. The whole process was very similar, if not identical, to the reconstructive surgery that a woman may undergo after a mastectomy.

My first surgery involved a saline implant. It was implanted empty and would be gradually filled over the following months, slowly stretching the skin to eventually match my left side. The doctor also created a new nipple, which I'm sure sounds funny, but was necessary. The implant would be expanded over time, stretching the skin closest to my armpit, thereby shifting what was already there to the left. Had he not shifted the location of my nipple, at the end of everything it would have been sideways, pointing to the left. I can still see where my original nipple was.

The procedure was done as an outpatient surgery and I was home the very same day. I was in tremendous pain in the days following, I think mainly due to an inaccurate dosage of pain medication. My arm was put in a sling to help me keep it and all the muscles on that side still. Any kind of movement or jostling caused pain. I sat up in bed that whole first day, sleeping in that position as well.

Getting comfortable was near impossible as even the slightest movement was painful. It was not a fun time. Between the pain and the vomiting from the pain medication, the following four to five days were miserable.

After a six-week recovery I began to have office visits every few weeks. My doctor would inject saline into the implant a little at a time. I don't recall the time frame here, but once he was content with the expansion it was time for another surgery. This time the permanent implant was put in. The subsequent surgeries were intended to improve the appearance of my right breast for symmetry.

There is still an obvious difference between my two sides, and I suspect more could have been done to fix that. However, after the surgery during my freshman year in college I decided I was done, and stopped going to any follow up appointments. It was good enough and I was content to move on.

Questions to Ask

If you are a parent of a daughter with PS, or you are a female with PS, you need to think about and discuss the options.

Allow your daughter to be part of the decision making process here. If you have done a good job up to this point in keeping PS an open topic of conversation, then I suspect the transition into this phase will not be too difficult.

I still have second thoughts about whether getting the surgeries was the right decision. Sure, it's nice to have a normal looking bust, but I am still lopsided since I cut my treatment short. I don't know if others notice, no one has ever said anything, although I don't know how one would broach such a topic anyway.

I sometimes wonder whether I'm denying who I am by having had the surgery. Since the surgery I had is very similar to that which women undergo after a mastectomy, I will sometimes ask myself, "If I had breast cancer, and had a mastectomy, would I want this surgery? Or would I accept my body as is?"

For me, these questions are largely a moot point, since I have had the surgery. I bring it up only to give you something to think about as you move forward and make these decisions.

Mom and dad, before you talk with your daughter, talk to each other about it. Talk about it from male and female perspectives. I always wondered how any man could want someone with an abnormal breast, only to discover that my husband couldn't care less. He loves me, scars and all. This will likely be a legitimate concern of your daughter.

Mom, bring up issues that you think may be issues. Dad, honestly give the male perspective, even if it's ugly. It's important that the two of you have a very honest dialogue about this so that you each understand the other's perspective before you address this with your daughter.

Then you do need to talk with her. Allow her to do much of the talking. It doesn't have to be a one-time talk. It may very well be a recurring discussion over the preteen years as she approaches adolescence. Allow her to express her opinions without your judgments. Don't tell her she is wrong, at least not yet.

If this is an ongoing talk in your home, there is no hurry. She may change her perspective one year to another, even one month to another. Give her the space to work through this on her own. If you and your spouse have a strong opinion one way or the other, eventually you will need to have more definitive discussions, but even here, you need to allow your daughter to voice her opinion. You need to remember two things:

It is her life and her body, BUT

She is still young, and young brains do not always make wise grown up decisions.

If your daughter wants to delay, putting off surgery isn't the worst decision. Surgery can always be done later, but you cannot undo a surgery.

If you do decide to have the surgery, fight for your daughter. Your insurance company will likely have a list of reasons why this isn't covered: pre-existing condition, elective, cosmetic surgery, who knows what else. Don't give up. Find a doctor who will also plead the case. Keep fighting until they cover it. File every petition, every extension. It will be tiring and emotional, but unless you are in a position to write a check for the surgery without blinking, it's worth the battle.

As the insurance company fights you, don't allow your love for your child to turn into misplaced guilt, causing you to take on debt to fund the surgery. Yes, the surgery is important (if you decide to take that route), but it is not life threatening. There is no ticking time bomb forcing you to pay with money you don't have before a certain date. You can love your daughter AND make wise financial choices. Don't let *anyone* convince you that you don't really love her unless you are willing to take on debt to do this.

Looking Forward

There is one aspect of this decision that wasn't even the remotest thought on my mind when I was 16 years old. I knew I had PS. I knew that my right breast would likely not grow at all, and would therefore not function like a normal breast. But I never thought about what that 'normal function' was. It wasn't until I was pregnant with my first child that I gave it any thought.

We live in a culture that equates women's breasts with sex, when really women's breasts were primarily designed to be the source of nourishment for their babies. In the months leading up to my daughters' birth, I wondered if I would be able to breastfeed. I was in for a surprise in more than one way.

I had prepared myself for the likely fact that my right breast would not produce milk due to PS. I was ready for that. I wasn't ready, however, to face regret over surgery decisions that resulted in added difficulty feeding.

It turns out my right breast did produce milk. It became engorged, as is supposed to happen. I was caught by surprise when I felt that sensation on my right side, but once I realize that despite the presence of milk, the baby would not be able to access it, I was overcome with deep sorrow.

You see, in the surgeries, the doctor moved my nipple, remember? In doing so, he closed off the proper exit for the milk. So here I had this milk but it could not get out. Now, I do not know how much milk my right side produced. I don't know if it would have been a normal amount of milk, but I do know that milk was there.

I was told by the lactation consultant that the body often makes up for any deficit on one side, producing additional milk on the good side. That too may be true, but I will never know for sure. One of the surgeries involved a "lift" to my left side. This wasn't directly related to PS, but it improved the symmetry, since a reconstructed breast doesn't look the same as a natural breast. The doctor felt this was a wise decision, and being a teen who hated to talk about the whole topic, I said, "Okay." Well, in doing this, he cut around the areola, cutting through the nerves and ducts that participate in the lactation process. As a result, the amount of milk produced and/or accessible on my left side was severely reduced.

This whole issue was never mentioned in any of the pre or post-surgery appointments. After giving birth, I called the surgeon to ask about how the surgeries would effect my ability to breastfeed. His response was that I wouldn't be able to breastfeed on the right side, but I should be able to on the left.

I have no gripes against my doctor personally, but I'd be lying to say that I wasn't frustrated and disappointed that *he* did not receive better training, especially in his chosen field. How could he not know the possible effects of breast surgery on the ability to later breastfeed?

I spent the first six weeks of that baby's life crying half the time, longing to be able to nurse her like I ought. Thankfully, with my second and third babies, I had more success and was able to nurse on the left side, providing 30% to 50% of their nourishment for the first 9 months or so. After that point, my body could not at all keep up with their hunger levels. With each birth, there has been some sadness, yet and I am learning to release the guilt I feel over having done this to myself.

I share all this to encourage you to consider all aspects of the decision. Do the cosmetic benefits outweigh the potential loss of ability to breastfeed your babies down the road? I think the medical community can rely on *their* "facts" too much sometime, and forget that the human body is an amazing thing. My doctor was certain that since my right breast did not grow it would have no function. Well, I'll never know how much function it had, but I do know the doctor was wrong.

{ 6 }

Lessons I've Learned

People Don't Care – And It's a Good Thing

Time and time again I am both surprised and humbled, by just how little people think about my hand. You see, for someone with PS, the deformity is never forgotten. You may not be specifically thinking about it every moment of the day, but you never forget that you don't have a normal hand. Well, in my experience, the same is not true for others, including my own husband.

We were enjoying a quiet evening at home watching a show. I was munching on some snack while sitting on the couch and had asked my husband to bring me a glass of milk. He brought it over and extended his arm to hand it to me. I was in mid-munch, with a cookie in my left hand when he tried to do the pass off. He was half distracted with the show and didn't hear me when I said, "Wait a minute."

Over time I have become quite skilled at balancing things with my right hand. I cannot grasp like a person with a full hand, but I can rotate my hand to extend the palm upwards, and do a pretty good job of balancing and carrying various items. Had the hand-off been done slower, there wouldn't have been a problem, but with him distracted he let go before I had the chance to balance.

As you can guess, the milk spilt all over the couch. I began to cry. I was mortified, as this was just another reminder of my hand being different. Yet, in that moment, my husband didn't understand.

For a moment, he was annoyed at the mess, but that changed immediately when he saw me. Then he thought *I* was upset about the mess. For him, my hand is a non-issue – it always has been. In that instance, my hand was not on his mind.

When you hand another person a glass you extend it, they take it, and it's done. That's what he was expecting. This still amazes me; how he can "forget." This is the person that knows me best in this world. I am closer to him than I am to anyone else, as it should be. Yet, he is still removed from my condition, to a degree, in that it is not something he regularly thinks about. Another reminder that while PS is something that I cannot escape, it is not as big an issue for others as I think it might be.

Late to the Game

In college sports, there is something called pre-season, which is code name for, "Run-them-till-it-hurts." I played soccer at my alma mater and during the pre-season, after one of our workout sessions, a teammate and I rode our bikes to the bookstore on campus. We stopped to get something to drink on the way and as we were locking up our bikes my teammate comments that she hadn't noticed my hand before (implying that she just now noticed). It was at least a week into preseason. By now we had easily spent well over thirty hours together as a team, yet she just now noticed? I was shocked but also relieved as it became clear that my hand isn't that obvious to people.

It's Okay to Say "No I'm Not Okay."

One of the biggest lessons I learned through all of this almost makes all the struggle worth it. Growing up I was taught (mostly by trial and error) to bottle up struggles and get on with life. Asking for help seemed shameful. Admitting that I was struggling with anything, whether school or sports or just life in general, felt like a weakness. It wasn't until I had hit the bottom with nowhere to go, in pure desperation, that I turned to a select few friends. It was from one of these friends that I was given this golden nugget of advice: "It's okay to say, 'No, I'm not okay.'"

When someone asks me, "How are you?" I could choose to be truthful instead of putting on my fake smile and playing the part of "Mel, who has it all together." What a thought!? Such honesty truly had never occurred to me before. "I'm good" seemed like the only proper response to that question. And answering in any other way seemed risky. But I began to try it anyway.

I played soccer my freshman year and quit at the end of the season. So the teammates I used to see for hours each day were no longer part of my daily routine. Our lives were simply lived in different spheres most of the time now. So when we crossed paths on campus, we'd usually take a few minutes to catch up. "How are you?" "What have you been up to?' "What's going on?' All typical questions from folks who really did care to know.

So often in our culture, we throw out, "How ya doing?" as a proper social grace, not really wanting an answer to the question. But I knew a handful of folks who, when they asked me that question, preferred an honest answer to a false one. So, I tried it.

The very next day, bright and early, I crossed paths with a former teammate as I was leaving the gym and she was entering. She asked how I was doing and I conveyed to her that I was struggling. She immediately asked if I wanted to get together later that day to talk about it, and we did.

After meeting up at the campus coffee shop I returned to my dorm walking on cloud nine. My problems didn't go away, but I was amazed, encouraged, and hopeful knowing that I had a friend who cared enough to meet up with me, on little notice, to listen to me babble on about my life. And she did listen. And she encouraged. And she thanked me for sharing. And it was helpful.

That very same week, maybe even that same day, I crossed paths with another soccer friend. This was actually the person I had in mind when I had decided to tell someone about my PS. Lo and behold, the opportunity arose. She opened the conversation saying, "Hey Mel, how are you?" Instead of giving my staged smile and false answer, I simply replied, "I'm okay." Which was as truthful an answer I had ever given to that question. Being the friend she is, able to read me, she asked, "Just okay?"

I had the choice to brush it off, and say, "No no, I'm good. Things are great." But instead I did what was most uncomfortable. I said, "Yeah, just okay." She pulled a bit more and I shared a little of the struggles I was having since quitting soccer, now dealing with issues that I had suppressed for so long, under my soccer life. We spoke for a few minutes, and then planned to meet up again to talk some more.

Even after having made that first step, it still wasn't easy to talk. But she persisted in the most loving way possible. "Talk to me Mel" was all she had to say to get me to relax and help me to open up. She would use that line more than once over the next three years. Whenever I'd clam up, not knowing where to start or what to say, I'd hear, "Just talk to me Mel" and somehow the words appeared.

She also taught me related lesson…

It's Not Complaining

Who can stand those folks who are always yapping about how bad their life is? Whining about this thing that happened, or what so-and-so said to them? Whiners. Complainers. Always looking for others to join their pity party. I cannot stand those folks and did not want to be one of them. One of the reasons I had avoided sharing my struggles with anyone for so long is that I "didn't want to complain." After all, my plight in life really ain't that bad. Sure, I have some physical deformities which cause some social embarrassment and some difficulties in day-to-day life, but I wasn't dying. I did not contract some terminal illness. I wasn't born with some chronic health condition. What was I complaining about? At least that is how I saw it.

When the aforementioned friend and I first sat down to talk I was largely apologetic for even bringing anything up because, "I didn't want to complain." But she responded, telling me that 'It isn't complaining, especially from you Mel." Now, maybe you are a complainer. Maybe you like to whine and get others to feel sorry for you. If that is the case, then it is whining, and you need to stop. But I suspect you are more like me, and you want to get on with life, but also deal with your struggles.

Perhaps you just don't know how to get on with life and need some help. If the latter better describes you, then it isn't complaining. Asking a friend for help isn't complaining. Telling a friend, "Hey, I'm struggling here, can you lend an ear?" isn't complaining. That is just what friends do. Life is hard, no matter who you are and situations will arise that we cannot handle on our own. It is okay to ask for help, and doing so isn't complaining. Whew. What a relief that was.

When Dealing with PS, I Don't Have to Appease Everyone

While I was at UPenn, I utilized their campus counseling service. It was a HUGE step for me and I am so glad that I did. I went for about 7 months, once a week. In one session we were dealing with my aversion to shaking hands. I was explaining my thought process as I entered into social settings and shook hands with people.

I shared with her the three types of people that I mentioned earlier. When I encounter the jumpers, I often reply, "That's okay" to lessen the embarrassment on their part because I can see their uneasiness with having just made a fool of themselves. But really, it didn't feel okay to me, because they embarrassed me as well.

Amy, my counselor, helped me realize that I did not have to take on the responsibility of easing their discomfort. I didn't have to make these people feel better. I could focus on what was best for me. It wasn't about being selfishness, but rather my misplaced, self-imposed role of making other people comfortable when I was not comfortable.

Why did I feel the need to say anything? Why tell them, "It's okay," when it's not. It goes back to being honest and not saying, "I'm good," when in truth, I'm not doing so well. Amy gave me permission to think about what made me feel most comfortable in these situations rather than what made others feel most comfortable.

It's a Process

All in all, I've come to realize that dealing with PS is a process and that baby steps are moving me in the right direction. I don't think I'll ever be completely comfortable in my own skin. There will always be a new challenge. With three kids every day presents a new challenge, even in the most mundane ways. Changing a newborn's messy diaper with 1 ½ hands. Learning how to put my own hair in a ponytail was challenging, but putting my girl's hair in ponytails is even more challenging. Life isn't getting any easier, and I have come to terms with that. As long as I am pressing forward, I know I am making progress.

I grew up on Long Island, NY. Summers were largely spent at one of the ocean beaches in the area, where the waves were constant. If you wanted to get out into the water, you had to first get past the waves. If you were timid and hesitant, you would either spend the day on the sand or get caught in an undertow. Neither was a very pleasant option. The only way to get past the whitewater was to dive in or dive over. You literally had to dive into (and through) the wave, or dive over it. Once you did that, you could enjoy the water, and even ride some waves back in.

Every day I wake up and am faced with waves of one kind or another. When I stand timid, I get caught in the undertow, leaving me frustrated. But when I dive in and face the challenge, I enjoy the satisfaction of accomplishing something hard. I increase my determination and perseverance. And I get to enjoy the "waves of life" that can be fun and quite adventurous, with three kids.

I have a choice as to the legacy I leave my kids. They can see their mom always frustrated, defeated by life and the hand (pun intended) she was dealt. Or they can see Mom living life, without much regard to her condition. They can see Mom accomplishing things that are difficult, yet not complaining. And hopefully they will be encouraged to hit the water head on. It's a choice I make every day. And while I wish I could snap my fingers and make it easy in an instant, I know that it is a life long process.

{ 7 }

Why me, God?

I remember lying on my bed as a kid, looking up at the ceiling in the dark of the night, crying out, "Why me, God, why me?" In total desperation and despair I pleaded to know why this happened to me. I saw nothing good in having been born with PS and there were challenges each and every day. Never would I be able to escape the effects of having PS. I was often miserable with myself and with life. Life felt pointless and my motto was "Life sucks and then you die."

As I went off to college my search for a purpose continued. I became an atheist, and though I studied a variety of religions in pursuit of life's meaning, my misery continued. As I mentioned earlier, after I quit soccer my freshman year I went into a depression, which continued for eighteen months. During that time, I had no regard for my life. I often "tempted fate" (as I called it), being careless in my daily life. Crossing streets without regard for city traffic. Going for a run at dusk in downtown Philadelphia –not the safest or smartest time to run. I just didn't care.

The way I saw my life, I was a pretty good person and this bad thing happened to me. It could be summed up in the question of "Why do bad things happen to good people?" I looked at myself compared to my peers and to my siblings. I went through a checklist of bad things I had never done, the good things I had done, and declared myself to be pretty darn good. So why would such a horrible thing (PS) happen to a good person like me? It was unfair.

During my final semester of college, after I got a handle on my depression, I was watching TV with a friend. Flipping through the channels we came across a "Where Are They Now" episode on the cast of Growing Pains. The actors talked about their experience on the show and what they have been doing since the show ended. When Kirk Cameron's turn came, he spoke about his family and a ministry called Way of the Master. He shared that, during the tail end of the show, he became a Christian.

This caught my attention. I had been studying all sorts of eastern religions, but had largely discounted Christianity. Having grown up attending a Lutheran Church, I had the perspective of, "Been there, done that." But here stood an attractive man, with fame and fortune, a beautiful wife and children. By the world's standards, he wasn't missing anything and yet he was a Christian. Intrigued, I went back to my dorm after the show, and Googled his name. What I encountered changed my life forever.

I came across his ministry website, and in flashing font (literally) was a link for a talk given by some guy with an Australian accent. In his message he spoke about the way men evaluate themselves compared to the way God evaluates them. For the first time, I realized that while I looked at my peers and said, "Well, I don't do this, or that, or that other thing, so I'm pretty good," God looked at me and says "Have you kept *all* of my laws?"

The speaker went through a few of the Ten Commandments, and as if he was talking directly to me, he asked, "Have you ever told a lie?" "Have you ever stolen anything in your life, regardless of its value?" "Have you ever used God's name as a cuss word to express disgust." He went on to explain that doing this was taking the name of the One who made me, and instead of giving that name honor, I was using it as a curse. He asked, "have you ever looked at another person with lust?' God says if you have looked with lust you have committed adultery in your heart. "Have you ever hated anyone?" If you hate your brother you are a murderer.

One by one, in the privacy of my dorm room, I admitted yes, yes, yes, yes and yes. I had done all of these things. I had told little white lies and big bold lies. I had stolen many things over the years. I thought nothing of using God's name as a curse. I had lusted after men more than once. And I had felt hatred towards many people over the course of my 21 years.

My situation wasn't looking too good. I felt ashamed and embarrassed. For the first time in my life I recognized that I wasn't a good person, not by a long shot! I was wicked. Really really wicked. My daily thoughts were cruel and perverse. I learned that there would be a day when I would stand before the God who made me and would have to give an account for everything I have said, done and thought. He would not compare me with others and grade on a curve. Instead, His test would be pass/fail, and my littlest white lie would lead to a failing grade. I was guilty and I knew it.

The just penalty for all this guilt would be an eternity in hell. You see, God cannot even look upon sin. He is holy and pure and just, and He will not allow sin into heaven, into His presence. All those who have broken His laws deserve to be punished, and I was one of them.

But, in the midst of this onslaught of guilt the man also shared some wonderful news. God is also merciful and kind, wanting to rescue us from hell. The man went on to explain something that I had never heard in all my years attending that Lutheran Church. Finally, someone explained why Jesus died on the cross. I knew the story; I knew it was for our sins, but I never really understood what that meant. This speaker provided an analogy that changed my life:

Imagine you are standing before a judge, guilty of the worse crimes you could imagine. You are guilty; the evidence is clear and abundant. There is no doubt in anyone's mind that you committed these crimes. The judge says to you, "You are guilty and there is a hefty fine to be paid. Your fine is $100,000,000,000. If you cannot pay, you will spend the rest of your life in prison."

You have no way to even begin to pay this fine, and so the bailiff steps forward to take you away. As he is taking you away, a stranger steps forward. You have never seen this man in your life, but he steps forward with a check in his hand and says, "Your Honor, I love this man, and I am here to pay his fine. I have sold all my earthly belongings so I could give you this. Here is a check for $100,000,000,000."

The speaker explained that with the fine paid, I was free to go. The law could no longer hold me. And my natural response to such an act would be tremendous gratitude to this stranger who freed me from the law. He went on to say that that stranger was Jesus Christ. I was guilty and Jesus paid my fine. It was as simple as that.

In Bible terms, if I would repent of my sins, which means turn from them, like I would turn my car around, and trust in His sacrifice on the cross, then God would forgive all my sins, past, present and future. If I would do that, God would actually give me a new heart, with new desires. Desires to love and obey Him whereas before I loved myself and obeyed my own selfish whims.

For the first time in my life, the cross made sense. I saw myself as that criminal before the judge, and was indeed so grateful for Jesus' willingness to pay my fine. Since that day, my life's purpose has been to bring God glory by obeying His Word and sharing His offer of salvation to anyone who will listen. My prayer is that someone out there, through reading this book, will also come to know His amazing love and find His forgiveness.

Forgiven for a Purpose

I did not wake up the next morning with my hand magically changed. I still have daily struggles with day-to-day activities. Neither has the Lord made me rich and powerful, like many televangelists claim will happen. God has done something even greater than all of that. He has given me the grace to get through each day. He has helped me to grow in patience and persistence. He has given me a compassion for others who struggle and is slowly replacing my pride with humility. But even if I never had another joyful day on this earth, He has saved me from hell. All of the earthly joys and comforts are such a small thing compared to the real prize of an eternity with God.

{ 8 }

Final Thoughts

Engaging Others

Children have a wonderful honesty. They often lack the *sophistication* of adults to hide what they are really thinking. I have found that most kids, once they notice my hand, have a hard time looking away. It often makes me laugh at first. Whether it's standing in line at the grocery store, or when I am coaching young soccer players, it's humorous to watch them try to adjust their position and viewing angle to get a look. Granted, my hand does looks strange, so it's natural to want to get a better look. I never mind their initial interest, but when it goes on for any length of time I will often begin to hide my hand in my jacket or pocket or the like. It can get annoying.

I have often thought about creating a plan to deal with such situations, broaching the subject for them so that they can see my hand without trying to "sneak-a-peek." But, being an introvert, I have yet to actually do this. In the meantime, I can offer a suggestion on how to prepare your own children (and maybe even yourself) to respectfully learn about other's disabilities.

You probably grew up being told, "It's not polite to stare," I know I was, and I'd agree. But that doesn't mean it cannot be talked about. I think there is a general misconception that those with deformities and the like just want to be left alone. I have found through interactions with others and my own experience, I would much rather someone say, "Hey, I noticed your hand, do you mind me asking what happened?" Instead, often in an attempt to be "respectful," we just stare.

I was in a store recently, in the checkout line to pay for my items. The cashier, in a very friendly and respectful tone said, "I'm sorry if this offends, but may I ask about your hand?" She was curious because she knows someone else with a hand similar to mine and was surprised at seeing a second such hand. It didn't offend at all, and I was happy to answer. Had she not asked and had she stared instead, I would have very much been offended and my own mindset upon leaving the store would not have been relaxed and appreciative of the question, but rather irritated and annoyed.

Another example, a woman in our church has some severe conditions that confine her to a wheelchair. She has no problem talking about her condition with those who inquire. In some ways the most respectful thing you can do is to ask. It shows respect for them as people and shows a desire to understand.

Granted, some people will not appreciate this. Some people will be offended and will react with anger. However, I suspect you would find that response in the minority of situations. If you approach the person in a humble manner, with a respectful tone, and with common sense (i.e. not interrupting their meal in a restaurant), I think you will find most people actually appreciate the opportunity to talk about their condition. And I think you may find a greater mutual respect is created when such conversations occur.

Going Forward

It is my prayer that as you finish this book you have a greater hope than when you started. If you are a parent, I pray that you are walking away with a greater understanding of your child and new tools to better help them thrive in their own lives. If you have PS, my prayer is that you will be strengthened in your resolve to succeed in life, unwilling to fall back upon your struggles as excuses.

Life is still lived one moment at a time, and each morning we are given a fresh start to make positive changes. May you be blessed by the reading of this book, and the resources listed at the end.

If this book impacted you in any way I would love to hear from you. You can reach me at
melissa@birthdefectpolandsyndrome.info

ABOUT THE AUTHOR

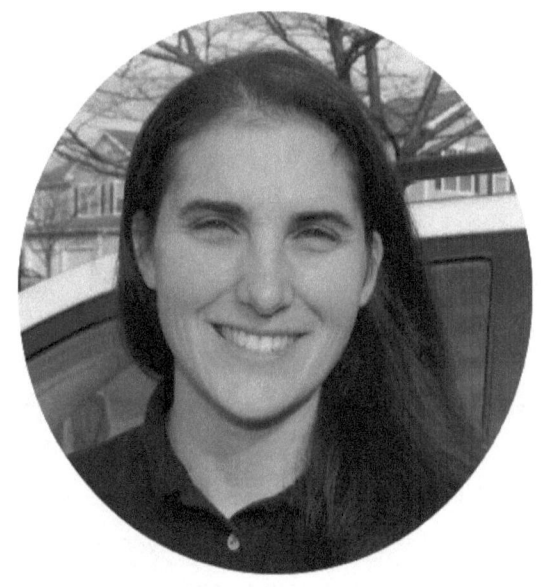

A New York transplant to rural Alabama, Melissa is a graduate of the Wharton School of the University of Pennsylvania. She holds a second degree black belt in IsshinRyu Karate, played Division 1 soccer at UPenn and currently homeschools her 4 children. You can follow Melissa at birthdefectpolandsyndrome.info and MelissaAmaya.com.

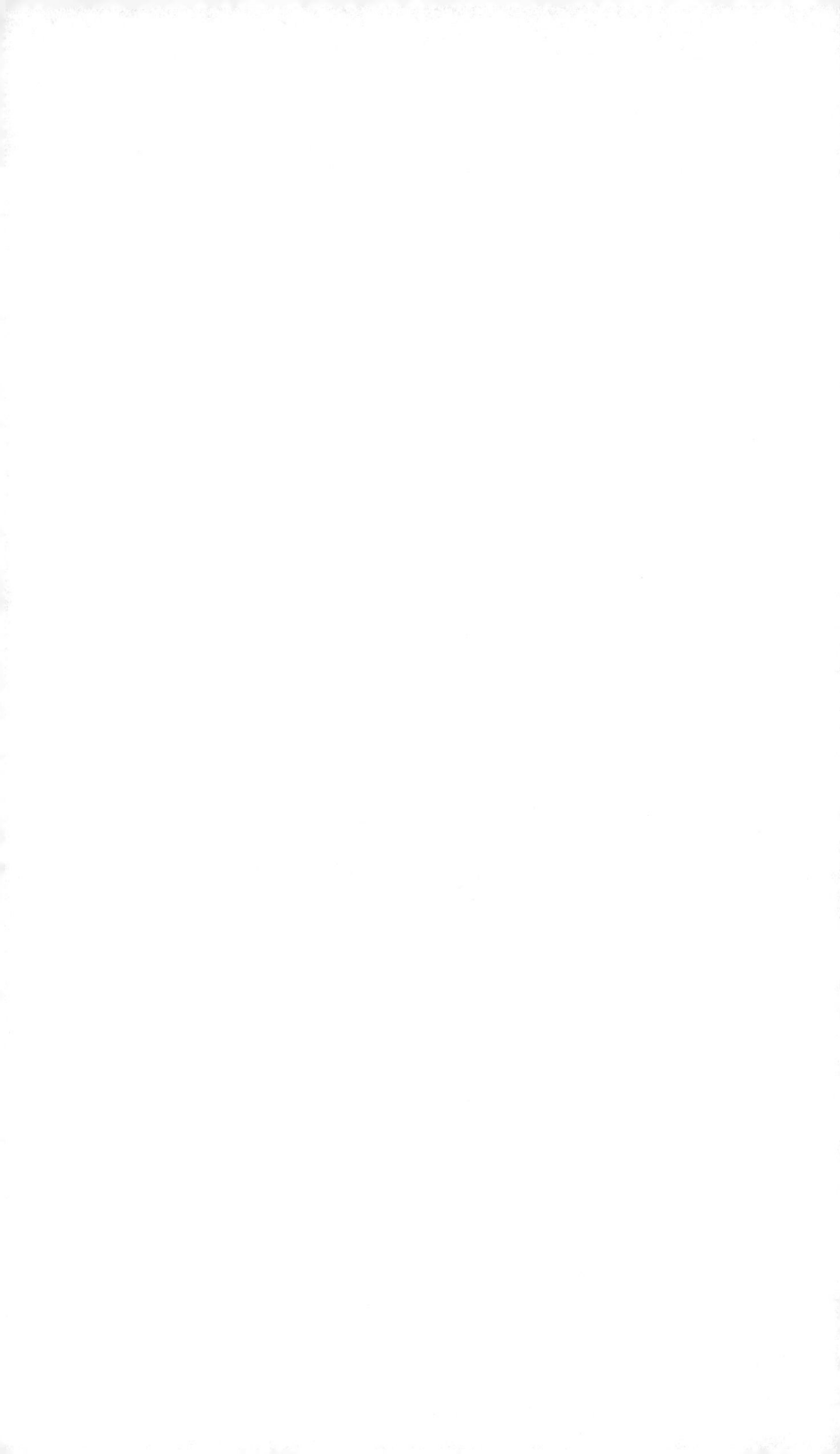

www.ingramcontent.com/pod-product-compliance
Lightning Source LLC
Chambersburg PA
CBHW030520290526
45786CB00004B/1544